# Pregnancy Journal

## and Memory Book

## With space for photos and memories

"A baby is God's opinion that life should go on."
~Carl Sandburg

A journal to document your
pregnancy as it happens!

"Having a baby is a life-changer. It gives you a whole other
perspective on why you wake up every day."
~Taylor Hanson

Find more unique, original baby books at babyfirstyearbooks.com
Baby memory books for your baby's first year of life.

*Mothers hold their children's hands for a short while,*
*but their hearts forever.*

# A New Baby

Having a baby is one of the most wonderful things that can happen to you. This pregnancy journal allows you to create a memory book and to monitor your pregnancy. You can document your thoughts, feelings, moods and cravings.

There are two pages of journal lines so you can write a letter to your baby plus additional pages so you can add a photo and write in special memories of your pregnancy.

Several additional pages available for memories include when you first learned you were pregnant, ultrasound photo page to how you and the baby's father met.

Other pages allow for keeping track of your pregnancy during each trimester. You can even add a photo that shows how you are changing as the baby grows.

Once your baby is born you can document the first moments of your baby's life, add photos and your baby's footprint.

The last section is for Autographs and Well-Wishes.

*A child's love could simply be one of the most beautiful sounds in the world.*

*A baby fills a place in your heart that you never knew was empty.*

"When you hold your baby in your arms the first time, and you think of all the things you can say and do to influence him, it's a tremendous responsibility.

What you do with him can influence not only him, but everyone he meets and not for a day or a month or a year, but for time and eternity."
~Rose Kennedy

# Happy Pregnancy Photo

Photo Here

Memories:

_____

_____

_____

_____

# I'm Pregnant!

What are some memories of the day you found out
you were having a baby?

_____

_____

_____

_____

_____

_____

_____

_____

Who was the first person you told?

_____

_____

_____

_____

What emotions did you feel?

_____

_____

_____

_____

_____

_____

# Letter To My Baby

_____

_____

_____

_____

_____

_____

_____

_____

_____

_____

# How Mommy and Daddy Met

There was a time before you were born when mommy and daddy first met. It was back in:

_____

_____

_____

_____

_____

The most memorable thing I remember was:

_____

_____

_____

_____

_____

# About Mommy

Name: _____

Date of Birth: _____

Place of Birth: _____

Favorite Things: _____

Favorite Food: _____

Favorite Music: _____

Favorite Color: _____

Special Memory: _____

_____

_____

_____

# About Daddy

Name: _____

Date of Birth: _____

Place of Birth: _____

Favorite Things: _____

Favorite Food: _____

Favorite Music: _____

Favorite Color: _____

Special Memory: _____

_____

_____

_____

# Our Family Tree

_____

Our Baby

_____     _____

_____     _____

_____     _____

Sisters                                          Brothers

_____     _____

Mommy                                          Daddy

_____     _____

Grandma                                        Grandma

_____     _____

Grandpa                                         Grandpa

*Every child is a different kind of flower, and all together make this world a beautiful garden.*

# Ultrasound

Photo Here

Date: _____

Memories of the day I had my ultrasound:

_____

_____

_____

_____

_____

_____

# Ultrasound

Photo Here

Date: _____

Memories of the day I had my ultrasound:

_____

_____

_____

_____

# First Trimester (0 to 13 Weeks)

# First Trimester Belly Photo

Photo Here

Date: _____

_____

_____

_____

_____

_____

# First Trimester Belly Photo

Photo Here

Date: _____

_____

_____

_____

_____

_____

# Week One

Date: _____

## How Am I Feeling

Mood: _____     Appetite: _____

Energy: _____     Cravings: _____

Morning Sickness: _____

## My thoughts and feelings:

_____

_____

_____

_____

_____

_____

_____

# Week Two

Date: _____

## How Am I Feeling

Mood: _____        Appetite: _____

Energy: _____        Cravings: _____

Morning Sickness: _____

**My thoughts and feelings:**

_____

_____

_____

_____

_____

_____

# Week Three

Date: _____

## How Am I Feeling

Mood: _____        Appetite: _____

Energy: _____        Cravings: _____

Morning Sickness: _____

## My thoughts and feelings:

_____

_____

_____

_____

_____

_____

# Week Four

Date: _____

## How Am I Feeling

Mood: _____    Appetite: _____

Energy: _____    Cravings: _____

Morning Sickness: _____

**My thoughts and feelings:**

_____

_____

_____

_____

_____

_____

_____

# Week Five

Date: _____

## How Am I Feeling

Mood: _____          Appetite: _____

Energy: _____          Cravings: _____

Morning Sickness: _____

## My thoughts and feelings:

_____

_____

_____

_____

_____

_____

# Week Six

Date: _____

## How Am I Feeling

Mood: _____     Appetite: _____

Energy: _____     Cravings: _____

Morning Sickness: _____

## My thoughts and feelings:

_____

_____

_____

_____

_____

_____

_____

# Week Seven

Date: _____

## How Am I Feeling

Mood: _____         Appetite: _____

Energy: _____        Cravings: _____

Morning Sickness: _____

**My thoughts and feelings:**

_____

_____

_____

_____

_____

_____

_____

# Week Eight

Date: _____

## How Am I Feeling

Mood: _____     Appetite: _____

Energy: _____     Cravings: _____

Morning Sickness: _____

**My thoughts and feelings:**

_____

_____

_____

_____

_____

_____

# Week Nine

Date: _____

## How Am I Feeling

Mood: _____     Appetite: _____

Energy: _____     Cravings: _____

Morning Sickness: _____

## My thoughts and feelings:

_____

_____

_____

_____

_____

_____

_____

# Week Ten

Date: _____

## How Am I Feeling

Mood: _____     Appetite: _____

Energy: _____     Cravings: _____

Morning Sickness: _____

## My thoughts and feelings:

_____

_____

_____

_____

_____

_____

# Week Eleven

Date: _____

## How Am I Feeling

Mood: _____     Appetite: _____

Energy: _____     Cravings: _____


Morning Sickness: _____


## My thoughts and feelings:

_____

_____

_____

_____

_____

_____

# Week Twelve

Date: _____

## How Am I Feeling

Mood: _____     Appetite: _____

Energy: _____     Cravings: _____

Morning Sickness: _____

## My thoughts and feelings:

_____

_____

_____

_____

_____

_____

# Week Thirteen

Date: _____

## How Am I Feeling

Mood: _____        Appetite: _____

Energy: _____        Cravings: _____

Morning Sickness: _____

## My thoughts and feelings:

_____

_____

_____

_____

_____

_____

## Additional Notes:

# Second Trimester (14 to 26 Weeks)

# Second Trimester Belly Photo

Photo Here

Date: _____

_____

_____

_____

_____

_____

# Second Trimester Belly Photo

Photo Here

Date: _____

_____

_____

_____

_____

_____

# Week Fourteen

Date: _____

## How Am I Feeling

Mood: _____          Appetite: _____

Energy: _____          Cravings: _____

Health/Sleep: _____

## My thoughts and feelings:

_____

_____

_____

_____

_____

_____

_____

# Week Fifthteen

Date: _____

## How Am I Feeling

Mood: _____          Appetite: _____

Energy: _____          Cravings: _____

Health/Sleep: _____

## My thoughts and feelings:

_____

_____

_____

_____

_____

_____

# Week Sixteen

Date: _____

## How Am I Feeling

Mood: _____    Appetite: _____

Energy: _____    Cravings: _____

Health/Sleep: _____

## My thoughts and feelings:

_____

_____

_____

_____

_____

_____

# Week Seventeen

Date: _____

## How Am I Feeling

Mood: _____     Appetite: _____

Energy: _____     Cravings: _____

Health/Sleep: _____

## My thoughts and feelings:

_____

_____

_____

_____

_____

_____

_____

# Week Eighteen

Date: _____

## How Am I Feeling

Mood: _____    Appetite: _____

Energy: _____    Cravings: _____

Health/Sleep: _____

## My thoughts and feelings:

_____

_____

_____

_____

_____

_____

_____

# Week Nineteen

Date: _____

## How Am I Feeling

Mood: _____　　Appetite: _____

Energy: _____　　Cravings: _____

Health/Sleep: _____

## My thoughts and feelings:

_____

_____

_____

_____

_____

_____

# Week Twenty

Date: _____

## How Am I Feeling

Mood: _____     Appetite: _____

Energy: _____     Cravings: _____

Health/Sleep: _____

## My thoughts and feelings:

_____

_____

_____

_____

_____

_____

# Week Twenty-one

Date: _____

## How Am I Feeling

Mood: _____     Appetite: _____

Energy: _____     Cravings: _____


Health/Sleep: _____

## My thoughts and feelings:

_____

_____

_____

_____

_____

_____

_____

# Week Twenty-two

Date: _____

## How Am I Feeling

Mood: _____     Appetite: _____

Energy: _____     Cravings: _____

Health/Sleep: _____

**My thoughts and feelings:**

_____

_____

_____

_____

_____

_____

_____

# Week Twenty-three

Date: _____

## How Am I Feeling

Mood: _____        Appetite: _____

Energy: _____        Cravings: _____

Health/Sleep: _____

## My thoughts and feelings:

_____

_____

_____

_____

_____

_____

# Week Twenty-four

Date: _____

## How Am I Feeling

Mood: _____          Appetite: _____

Energy: _____          Cravings: _____


Health/Sleep: _____


## My thoughts and feelings:

_____

_____

_____

_____

_____

_____

# Week Twenty-five

Date: _____

## How Am I Feeling

Mood: _____     Appetite: _____

Energy: _____     Cravings: _____

Health/Sleep: _____

## My thoughts and feelings:

_____

_____

_____

_____

_____

_____

# Week Twenty-six

Date: _____

## How Am I Feeling

Mood: _____          Appetite: _____

Energy: _____          Cravings: _____


Health/Sleep: _____

## My thoughts and feelings:

_____

_____

_____

_____

_____

_____

Additional Notes:

_____

_____

_____

_____

_____

_____

_____

_____

_____

_____

# Third Trimester (27 to 40 Weeks)

# Third Trimester Belly Photo

Photo Here

Date: _____

_____

_____

_____

_____

_____

# Third Trimester Belly Photo

Photo Here

Date: _____

_____

_____

_____

_____

_____

# Week Twenty-seven

Date: _____

## How Am I Feeling

Mood: _____     Appetite: _____

Energy: _____     Cravings: _____

Health/Sleep: _____

## My thoughts and feelings:

_____

_____

_____

_____

_____

_____

# Week Twenty-eight

Date: _____

## How Am I Feeling

Mood: _____     Appetite: _____

Energy: _____     Cravings: _____

Health/Sleep: _____

## My thoughts and feelings:

_____

_____

_____

_____

_____

_____

# Week Twenty-nine

Date: _____

## How Am I Feeling

Mood: _____     Appetite: _____

Energy: _____     Cravings: _____

Health/Sleep: _____

## My thoughts and feelings:

_____

_____

_____

_____

_____

_____

_____

# Week Thirty

Date: _____

## How Am I Feeling

Mood: _____     Appetite: _____

Energy: _____     Cravings: _____

Health/Sleep: _____

## My thoughts and feelings:

_____

_____

_____

_____

_____

_____

_____

# Week Thirty-one

Date: _____

## How Am I Feeling

Mood: _____     Appetite: _____

Energy: _____     Cravings: _____

Health/Sleep: _____

## My thoughts and feelings:

_____

_____

_____

_____

_____

_____

# Week Thirty-two

Date: _____

## How Am I Feeling

Mood: _____     Appetite: _____

Energy: _____     Cravings: _____

Health/Sleep: _____

## My thoughts and feelings:

_____

_____

_____

_____

_____

_____

_____

# Week Thirty-three

Date: _____

## How Am I Feeling

Mood: _____    Appetite: _____

Energy: _____    Cravings: _____

Health/Sleep: _____

**My thoughts and feelings:**

_____

_____

_____

_____

_____

_____

# Week Thirty-four

Date: _____

## How Am I Feeling

Mood: _____          Appetite: _____

Energy: _____          Cravings: _____

Health/Sleep: _____

## My thoughts and feelings:

_____

_____

_____

_____

_____

_____

_____

# Week Thirty-five

Date: _____

## How Am I Feeling

Mood: _____     Appetite: _____

Energy: _____     Cravings: _____

Health/Sleep: _____

**My thoughts and feelings:**

_____

_____

_____

_____

_____

_____

# Week Thirty-six

Date: _____

## How Am I Feeling

Mood: _____          Appetite: _____

Energy: _____          Cravings: _____


Health/Sleep: _____

## My thoughts and feelings:

_____

_____

_____

_____

_____

_____

_____

# Week Thirty-seven

Date: _____

## How Am I Feeling

Mood: _____        Appetite: _____

Energy: _____        Cravings: _____

Health/Sleep: _____

## My thoughts and feelings:

_____

_____

_____

_____

_____

_____

# Week Thirty-eight

Date: _____

## How Am I Feeling

Mood: _____     Appetite: _____

Energy: _____     Cravings: _____

Health/Sleep: _____

## My thoughts and feelings:

_____

_____

_____

_____

_____

_____

_____

# Week Thirty-nine

Date: _____

## How Am I Feeling

Mood: _____     Appetite: _____

Energy: _____     Cravings: _____

Health/Sleep: _____

## My thoughts and feelings:

_____

_____

_____

_____

_____

_____

# Week Forty

Date: _____

## How Am I Feeling

Mood: _____          Appetite: _____

Energy: _____          Cravings: _____


Health/Sleep: _____

## My thoughts and feelings:

_____

_____

_____

_____

_____

_____

_____

# Week Forty-one

Date: _____

## How Am I Feeling

Mood: _____          Appetite: _____

Energy: _____          Cravings: _____


Health/Sleep: _____


**My thoughts and feelings:**

_____

_____

_____

_____

_____

_____

_____

## Additional Notes:

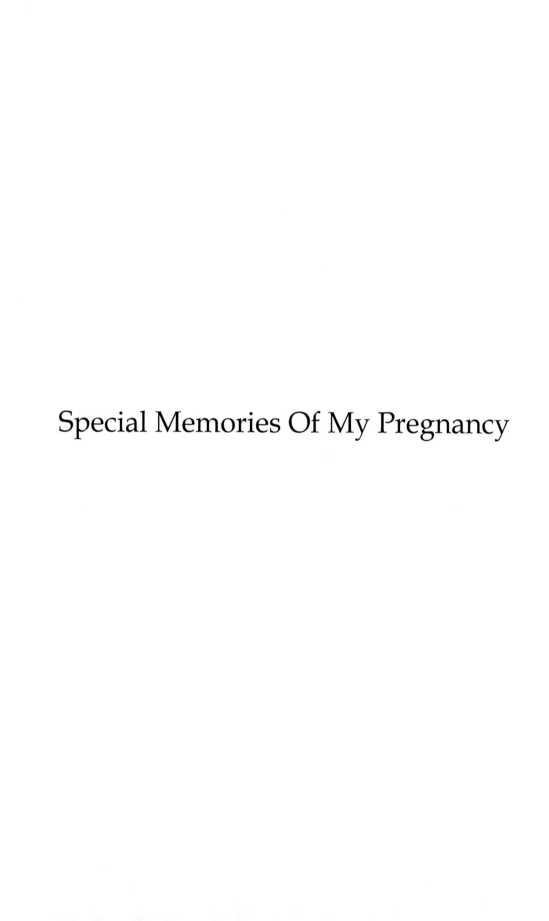

Special Memories Of My Pregnancy

# Memories:

Date: _____

```
+-------------------------------------+
|                                     |
|                                     |
|                                     |
|             Photo Here              |
|                                     |
|                                     |
|                                     |
|                                     |
+-------------------------------------+
```

_____

_____

_____

_____

_____

Date: _____

```
┌─────────────────────────────┐
│                             │
│                             │
│                             │
│         Photo Here          │
│                             │
│                             │
│                             │
│                             │
└─────────────────────────────┘
```

_____

_____

_____

_____

_____

Date: _____

Photo Here

_____

_____

_____

_____

_____

_____

Date: _____

Photo Here

_____

_____

_____

_____

_____

Date: _____

```
┌─────────────────────────────────┐
│                                 │
│                                 │
│                                 │
│          Photo Here             │
│                                 │
│                                 │
│                                 │
│                                 │
└─────────────────────────────────┘
```

_____

_____

_____

_____

_____

Date: _____

Photo Here

_____

_____

_____

_____

_____

Date: _____

Photo Here

_____

_____

_____

_____

_____

_____

Date: _____

```
┌─────────────────────────────────────┐
│                                      │
│                                      │
│                                      │
│              Photo Here              │
│                                      │
│                                      │
│                                      │
└─────────────────────────────────────┘
```

_____

_____

_____

_____

_____

Date: _____

Photo Here

_____

_____

_____

_____

_____

_____

Date: _____

Photo Here

_____

_____

_____

_____

_____

Date: _____

Photo Here

_____

_____

_____

_____

_____

_____

# Special Memories of Your Birth

Memories:

_____

_____

_____

_____

_____

_____

_____

_____

_____

_____

Memories:

_____

_____

_____

_____

_____

_____

_____

_____

_____

_____

# Welcome Baby
(The first time I touched you and saw your face)

# Birth Announcement

## Welcoming

_____

_____

```
┌─────────────────────────────────────┐
│                                     │
│                                     │
│                                     │
│              Photo Here             │
│                                     │
│                                     │
│                                     │
└─────────────────────────────────────┘
```

Date of Birth: _____

Time of Birth: _____

Birth Weight: _____

Date: _____

Photo Here

_____

_____

_____

_____

_____

_____

Date: _____

Photo Here

_____

_____

_____

_____

_____

Date: _____

```
┌─────────────────────────────────┐
│                                 │
│                                 │
│                                 │
│           Photo Here            │
│                                 │
│                                 │
│                                 │
└─────────────────────────────────┘
```

_____

_____

_____

_____

_____

Date: _____

Photo Here

_____

_____

_____

_____

_____

Date: _____

```
┌─────────────────────────────────┐
│                                 │
│                                 │
│                                 │
│          Photo Here             │
│                                 │
│                                 │
│                                 │
│                                 │
└─────────────────────────────────┘
```

_____

_____

_____

_____

_____

Date: _____

```
┌─────────────────────────────────────┐
│                                      │
│                                      │
│                                      │
│                                      │
│              Photo Here              │
│                                      │
│                                      │
│                                      │
│                                      │
└─────────────────────────────────────┘
```

_____

_____

_____

_____

_____

Date: _____

Photo Here

_____

_____

_____

_____

_____

Date: _____

Photo Here

_____

_____

_____

_____

_____

Date: _____

Photo Here

_____

_____

_____

_____

_____

_____

*The littlest feet make the biggest footprints in our hearts.*

# Baby Handprint & Footprint

# My Baby's Handprint

Date: _____

# My Baby's Footprint

Date: _____

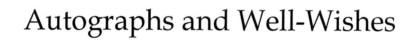
Autographs and Well-Wishes

# Autographs and Well-Wishes

# Autographs and Well-Wishes

# Autographs and Well-Wishes

# Autographs and Well-Wishes

# Autographs and Well-Wishes

# Autographs and Well-Wishes

CPSIA information can be obtained
at www.ICGtesting.com
Printed in the USA
FFOW01n2158161115
18723FF

9 781516 836079